Acid Reflux Diet

A Beginner's Guide To Natural Cures And Recipes For
Acid Reflux, GERD And Heartburn

By Susan T. Williams

FREE EBOOK: 101 SECRETS TO WEIGHT LOSS SUCCESS

available at

www.TheTotalEvolution.Com

Table of Contents

Introduction

Rumble, burp, ouch.

How often do you get those unbearable acid-filled hiccups? Have you been suffering from a searing abdominal pain that just wouldn't go away?

Or do you wake up in the middle of the night with a tightened throat or a terrifying sensation of choking?

Do you experience debilitating stomach cramps?

When you have to live with symptoms like these, life is nothing short of abject misery. And no, don't worry, you are not alone.

Acid reflux, or GERD (gastro esophageal reflux disease) as its commonly called these days, is a common digestive disorder. It is a chronic recurrent condition that affects millions of Americans. Yet, many of them are not well informed about it.

In "Acid Reflux Diet: A Beginner's Guide To Natural Cures And Recipes For Acid Reflux, GERD And Heartburn", we outline a cooking and lifestyle plan you can rely on to manage and cure GERD symptoms. The book recommends snacks and meals you can dig into with delight without worrying about acid reflux. It also warns against food items which will cause flare-ups. If you think living with Acid Reflux means depriving yourself of all your favorite food items, you are in for a surprise.

This eBook is ideally suitable for you if you are:

• Suffering from heartburn • Looking for healthy acid reflux diet recipes • Looking for a beginner's cookbook for GERD-friendly recipes• Seeking a natural cure and relief from heartburn and GERD symptoms • Looking for delicious diet recipes • Looking for tasty low-fat recipes

This book will be your quintessential guide to living a healthier and happier life with GERD by safely eliminating the causes of acid reflux and ensuring relief from its symptoms. Remember, GERD symptoms do not disappear by popping antacids like candy.

The first part of this book deals primarily with the technical aspects of GERD and gives you clear background information and doable lifestyle changes to help manage it.

The second part of the book outlines how transitioning to a GERD Diet can reduce the amount of stress that's placed on your system, effectively controlling and combating Acid Reflux. We also cover all the main food items you should exclude and banish from your diet so you can effectively treat the condition and even free yourself from GERD symptoms.

By staying consistent with your efforts and ensuring that the wrong food items don't enter your system, you will start to see significant improvements almost immediately.

We saved the best for last.

"Acid Reflux Diet: A Beginner's Guide To Natural Cures And Recipes For Acid Reflux, GERD And Heartburn" includes healthy GERD and acid reflux diet recipes which will allow you to naturally prevent both disorders—starting with breakfast all the way to dinner. Most of the ingredients for these sumptuous recipes may already be available in your refrigerator or on your kitchen shelves.

This book will take you back to the time when eating was joy, without any discomfort or fear accompanying it. Imagine enjoying a meal without worry or discomfort.

When you follow a GERD friendly lifestyle, you will also shed some unwanted fat, reduce your chances of developing other inflammatory illnesses like cancer and diabetes and experience overall good health.

If you thought you were doomed to a life of suffering, and a diet of water and crackers this book will help you to banish the bland and start eating your way to a wonderful, healthy life without Acid Reflux.

CHAPTER 1

Your food could be eating your insides

Listen closely; your stomach may be burning to tell you something.

For you, it's just another day full of deadlines. It's a crazy day that began with coffee and chaos. Lunch time is unthinkable because you have absolutely no time for lunch. But your stomach doesn't know any better. It grumbles—loudly. Quickly, you reach for the pack of Twinkies to ease your hunger. Soon, all you can think about is the hot, burning feeling that rises up from your stomach. Could it be stomach acid making its way up to your heart?

Heartburn, thankfully, does not have anything to do with your heart.

But it has everything to do with the food you swallowed and how it moves through your esophagus and makes its way smoothly down into your stomach.

The lower esophageal sphincter (LES), a muscle that connects the esophagus and the stomach, acts like a security gate or "one way valve". It usually only allows food to enter into the stomach and then it closes again. Your stomach does its part and secretes bile and digestive juices, which break down food. The sphincter keeps the food and acidic stomach juices from flowing back into the esophagus.

If the LES is weakened, or does not close properly, this causes semi-digested food and caustic gastric acids to go back up into the esophagus, resulting in gastro esophageal reflux. The esophagus gets irritated when acidic content from the stomach comes back up, and this process is what causes a burning sensation.

Acid Reflux can cause your quality of life to deteriorate.

The stomach is smartly designed to handle the strong gastric juices required to digest food. The esophagus, however, just cannot tolerate them. Stomach acids contain hydrochloric acids and enzymes which have a highly corrosive quality.

When you think of hydrochloric acids, you instantly think of a strong acid that is used in a wide range of industrial processes, one that can cause your skin to burn if there is contact. You think of anti-corrosive and well-sealed containers with bright danger signs pasted on them. If your skin is exposed to hydrochloric acids, it can even cause severe chemical burns. Can you then imagine what kind of damage could be caused to the tender lining of the esophagus by repeated exposure to such acids?

Other than the discomfort it causes you, GERD also harms the esophagus over time. Sometimes, untreated chronic GERD can even trigger several other complications ranging from inflammation to open sores and scarring. GERD can also cause changes to the cells lining the esophagus. Changes in these cells raise the risk of esophageal cancer.

Living with GERD may not be easy. There will be times when you are angry at the situation. You feel great when you don't eat and the moment you swallow something, the discomfort starts. Eating shouldn't be this stressful because it is truly one of the greater pleasures in life.

Your friends and family may think you are exaggerating about your symptoms and that you should lighten up about your heartburn. It is after all, not like you were diagnosed with a terminal disease. But dealing with the constant chest pain, the constant meal planning and and the fatigue from sleeplessness and pain can really bring you down.

Acid Reflux is preventable.

Healthy lifestyle changes and avoiding all the food items that exacerbate your symptoms can be very helpful in alleviating the discomfort caused by acid reflux. As you read on, you will find out how you can lead a healthy life, and enjoy food items you love—even with Acid Reflux. And what you find on the menu of recommended foods may surprise you greatly.

CHAPTER 2

Do you have the Acid Reflux blues?

Acid Reflux associated symptoms

While the symptoms vary from person to person, if you answer "yes" to one or more of the following, you may be experiencing symptoms of acid reflux. Sure, the severity level may be different, but please do not ignore any symptoms, even if you think they are not important.

1. Do you frequently experience heartburn, a burning sensation in your chest and/or throat? Do you have a sour or acidic taste in your mouth?

2. Do you have difficulty swallowing? Is swallowing painful?

This may be due to damage caused to the lining of your esophagus by exposure to stomach acids. When the damage heals it forms scar tissue. As a result, the esophagus becomes narrow, and you find it hard to swallow.

3. Do you have a dry cough?

Sometimes, dry cough and asthma-like symptoms are often mistaken for allergies. If you have a persistent dry cough, it is a good idea to have it checked by a medical professional.

4. Do you have sore throat that makes you sound hoarse?

Acid Reflux affects the throat and larynx. An inflammation in this area results in a sore throat and/or hoarse voice.

5. Do you often notice any swallowed food or sour-tasting contents of your stomach coming back into your mouth?

6. Do you feel like you have a lump in your throat?

7. Have you experienced bleeding?

An esophageal ulcer caused by the erosion of the walls of the esophagus by stomach acid can cause an open sore, which can occasionally bleed.

8. Do you have chest pains?

9. Are your teeth and gums getting eroded by the stomach acids that reach your mouth?

10. Do you experience difficulty in breathing?

CHAPTER 3

The Unsettling reality of life with Acid Reflux

Conventional medication works to block or neutralize acid production in the stomach. Acid-inhibiting medications such as proton pump inhibitors or H(2)-receptors block the stomach's production of acid. Prolonged use of these may cause a state of chronic low acid in your stomach resulting in improperly digested food.

And once you stop the meds, acid indigestion may recur. Medication does not provide a long term solution because it does not address the root causes of Acid Reflux. Prescription medication is not the answer to GERD unless you are willing to count on a lifelong dependency on pharmaceutical products as a solution for your problems. It may be a short-term fix that may actually exacerbate the problem over time because you only mask your symptoms.

Get to the bottom of what is causing your Acid Reflux.

The cause could be something very simple. Anything could trigger Acid Reflux—from something that you eat, to your lifestyle, to even the bacteria residing in your gut. Let's take a look at some of the things that could be causing your symptoms.

Food—processed, fatty, fried or spicy food, dairy, citrus food, tomatoes

Alcohol

Caffeine

Smoking

Eating too fast

Eating right before bed

Overeating

Being overweight. Extra pounds around your gut push your stomach up, causing acid to back up into your esophagus.

Chronic stress. Your stomach nerves are affected and this prevents proper digestion of food

Dairy, gluten and sugar sensitivities

Presence of bad bacteria or yeast in your stomach caused by consumption of excessive sugar and processed food, antibiotics, hormones. These bacteria ferment and move things around your gut, resulting in reflux.

A bacterium called H. Pylori

CHAPTER 4

Suffering from acid reflux is simply unnecessary.

How would you react if I were to tell you that there is a way you can be in control of your heartburn and acid reflux symptoms? Yes. It's easy. All you have to do is make a few changes to your diet and your lifestyle, and you can regain control of your life and overcome GERD symptoms.

GERD does not go away, but you are able to alleviate and in many cases, prevent the painful symptoms. We are all unique individuals, so the path back to where your Acid Reflux began can be different for everyone.

Get a grip on your GERD. Here are some tips and tricks on how.

Your food: There is no absolute eat-this-not-that list, but mindful eating and the following pointers may help you in avoiding heartburn.

The size of your meals.

Eat smaller portions. When you overeat, gastric pressure is built up in your stomach, and puts extra strain on the lower esophageal sphincter (LES), which could cause food to move back into the esophagus from the stomach. Eat small meals, and eat more frequently.

Almost everyone likes Italian food, so why not eat like Italian people? Research shows that Italians experience less Acid Reflux symptoms in comparison to people in the United States. Could it could be the smaller portion sizes they eat? Or could it be the smaller amount of sauce that accompanies the pasta in their plates? Or perhaps the fact that they include a side dish of vegetables at all meals? Well, the answer to all the questions is YES.

Eat slowly.

Yes, you have that deadline fast-approaching. Perhaps, you are running late for a client meeting.

So, you grab, gobble and go. If you want to tame your heartburn, wolfing down food is an absolute no-no. Chew slowly; allow the saliva in your mouth to mix thoroughly with the food. Slow down, breathe and enjoy an unhurried meal.

Only go to sleep a minimum of 2-3 hours after a meal.

When you lay down with a full stomach, you are increasing the chances that the contents of your stomach will move back into the esophagus and cause heartburn.

Method of preparation

Food preparation methods matter. As a rule, avoid all fried food. Roasting, grilling, steaming or poaching are better options.

Keep it simple.

Avoid too great a variety in a given meal. Your stomach will protest if you eat more than three or four dishes at mealtime.

Don't consume food which triggers heartburn.

Several food items and beverages are known to trigger heartburn. They either increase acid production and gastric pressure or make the sphincter muscle loose. Some kinds of food irritate the lining of the esophagus, such as the ones listed below:

Fried, spicy or fatty food
Citrus fruits and juices
Chocolate
Peppermint or spearmint
Garlic
Chili pepper
Onions
Tomato
Coffee
Caffeinated Tea and Soft Drinks
Alcoholic Beverages
Dairy

Eating any of these food items for dinner can cause Acid Reflux at night. Initially, you may not be sure of what kinds of food trigger your heartburn. Raw green peppers may suit your friend, but may cause a riot in your stomach.

Keep a food diary for ten days. Make note of how you feel after eating different kinds of food. Soon, you will find a clear pattern emerging.

High-fat meals don't do you any good.

Gorging on high-fat food items only result in excess weight gain and an increased risk of acid reflux symptoms. Fried and fatty food items are known to weaken the lower esophageal sphincter (LES), thus allowing stomach content into the esophagus. Most people love fried food, and therefore it's very easy to overeat fried delicacies.

Try a low-carb diet.

A diet rich in high-carbohydrate food causes your digestive system to become overloaded while attempting to break down the food. When carbohydrates are not absorbed properly in the small intestine, it can result in the growth of bacteria, which can cause excessive gas in your bowels. The gas puts excess pressure on the upper digestive system, and that causes Acid Reflux. Adopt a low glycemic diet to avoid heartburn. However, stay away from the processed low-carb food items sold in supermarkets. Instead, consume more wholesome, real food items that are low carb.

Maintain an upright posture.

Don't slouch after a meal. Standing or sitting straight facilitates proper digestion. A short walk or a spot of yoga does wonders for your digestion as well. The Thunder Bolt Pose or Vajrasana helps to increase the blood flow to the stomach and to digest food effectively. It's very easy to perform as well. Sit straight on your knees, with your bottom touching your heels. Rest your hands on the knees. Keep your head straight. Breathe naturally and stay in this pose for 5 – 10 minutes.

Left-side sleeping helps.

The lower esophageal sphincter (LES) is located on the left side of your stomach. If it is weak, and doesn't close properly, sleeping on your right side may cause the acidic contents of your stomach to go backwards into the esophagus. Over time, this can cause damage to the lining of the esophagus and cause you pain.

Avoid the consumption of alcohol.

Alcohol can cause damage in two ways, so it is advisable to stop or reduce consumption if you are suffering from Acid Reflux. First, it increases the acid production in your stomach and second, it can relax your lower esophageal sphincter (LES). When the sphincter is not doing its job, the stomach acids flow back into the esophagus, thus increasing your heartburn.

No Smoking.

Acid reflux gives you another reason to stop smoking. When you inhale smoke, the production of stomach acids gets stimulated. The lower esophageal sphincter (LES)'s ability to function properly is also reduced.

Antacids or heartburn helpers help.

Pickles, lozenges and chewing gum are heartburn helpers that help to activate the production of saliva which aids in the digestive process.

If you are in extreme discomfort, reach for an antacid. They can provide quick relief. A medical professional may recommend H(2) blockers which work for a longer time, or a proton pump inhibitor for acute cases.

Keep your head at a higher level than your body when you sleep.

This is easy to understand. When your head and shoulders are at a higher level, the contents in your stomach have no way of flowing upwards into the esophagus. You could either get a wedge shaped pillow to raise our head, or position two pillows at the head board of your bed at an angle. Another way is to elevate the entire bed by placing sturdy bricks or blocks under the legs of the bed on the side you place your head.

Avoid wearing tight clothes.

Wearing clothes that are tight around your mid-section will press against your stomach and force food against the lower esophageal sphincter (LES), and reflux into your esophagus. Try not to wear tight belts and slimming body suits, Spanx and undergarments which squeeze your stomach.

Overweight? Try to maintain a healthy weight.

Extra weight puts pressure on your stomach by pushing it up and results in stomach acids backing up into the esophagus. If you are overweight or obese, try to lose some of the extra weight, but work slowly and purposefully towards your weight goal. Do not fast track your weight loss by following a fad diet.

Relax.

You may find your Acid Reflux symptoms acting up at all the wrong times—such as when you have a job interview or when your performance review is due. You may be under great stress, and your heartburn doesn't improve the situation. Though there aren't any direct links between heartburn and stress, many studies have concluded that when you are in stressful situations, you are more sensitive to stomach acids in the esophagus. Being under stress may reduce the production of "prostaglandins," a substance which protects the stomach from the effects of acid, and that could be why you have a heightened sense of discomfort.

CHAPTER 5

Getting started with the Acid Reflux Diet

The discomfort and complications caused by acid reflux and heartburn can potentially affect every area of your day-to-day life. Finding the right treatment is often a step-by-step process which involves trial and error. What works for you may be ineffective for someone else.

The Acid Reflux Diet is all about making changes to your life and the way you think.

It's about wanting to feel better and becoming healthier.

It's about transforming how food influences you.

It's about reducing the intake of food items that produce the most acid.

It's about avoiding food items that relax the lower esophageal sphincter (LES).

It's about planning on when and how much you eat in order to minimize heartburn.

And mostly, it's about preparing delicious, easy menus and trying out different recipes to support your changed eating habits.

An Acid Reflux diet, in combination with the other lifestyle changes we have discussed in the previous chapters, can often help reduce, or even eliminate many of the painful symptoms associated with this condition.

The best place to start would be to gain a clear understanding of what Acid Reflux is. Find out its causes, symptoms and how it affects your body. The next step would be to observe carefully how your body responds to specific food items. All these steps are essential to help you work out a diet plan to manage your GERD.

A pinch of patience, a dash of creativity and a spoonful of experimentation.

For many years, studies in the area of acid reflux and GERD have revealed many new developments.

However, one thing that is evergreen is that there is no "one size fits all" cure or diet for everyone. Each person is different and shows different symptoms and reactions to different food and treatment options. Therefore it is important that you modify and customize your eating and lifestyle habits accordingly.

Different food choices for different folks?

As there is no definitive Acid Reflux diet that works in all circumstances, you may need to invest time to patiently work out an Acid Reflux diet that works for you. You can choose from a great variety food items that have been known to treat heartburn symptoms and encourage your body to heal itself.

Start with an elimination diet. You will be able to find out if a certain food or food group is causing heartburn symptoms or making it exacerbate.

An elimination diet can be divided into four different steps.

Create an action plan.

You could either work on creating an action plan alone or seek your medical practitioner's assistance. Get to know which food items could cause your heartburn to flare up. Maintain a diet journal. List all the food items you eat during the entire week and mark the symptoms you have experienced after consumption of these food items.

Here is an example of what your 7-day food chart would look like.

7-DAY FOOD CHART (INCLUDE FOOD ITEMS EATEN AND AT WHAT TIMES. NOTE THE SYMPTOMS YOU EXPERIENCE AND AT WHAT TIME)							
	DAY 1	DAY 2	DAY 3	DAY 4	DAY 5	DAY 6	DAY 7
MORNING MEAL							
MORNING SYMPTOM							
AFTERNOON MEAL							
AFTERNOON SYMPTOM							
EVENING MEAL							
EVENING SYMPTOM							

Compare the food items in the chart with the following list:

Food items you eat often.

Food you crave.

Food items you eat for relief from heartburn.

Food items you find hard to resist.

Below is a list of food and beverages that may increase your heartburn symptoms.

Food group	Preferred food items	Food offenders
Fish, poultry, meat	Fish, chicken, turkey, lamb	Eggs, red meat, processed meat
Fats/oils	Flax, refined olive oils, pumpkin, sesame and walnut oils	Margarine, shortening, butter, and spreads, fried food items
Dairy	Rice milk, soy and nut milks like almond milk	Cow's milk, cheese, ice cream, yogurt
Fruits	Fresh or juiced	Citrus fruits
Beverages	Drinking water, herbal teas, fresh and unsweetened fruit/ vegetable juices	Alcohol, coffee, chocolate, tea, sodas, tomato juice, citrus juices
Sweeteners	Brown rice syrup, dates, fruit sweeteners	Honey, brown sugar, fructose, molasses

The avoiding phase

During the second and third week, you eliminate the food items that cause you heartburn symptoms entirely from your diet. Take care you don't consume these food items at all. Avoid them even in small portions.

For instance, if you are avoiding eggs, you need to check the labels on processed or packaged food items for ingredients like albumin, flavoprotein, globulin, livetin or ovalbuman so you can avoid any food that has traces of eggs in it. Sauces like béarnaise sauce, mayonnaise, hollandaise sauce and meringue also contain eggs, so it's best to stay away from foods containing these ingredients.

It's true that you need to be extremely disciplined when you are going through this phase of the elimination diet. Be ever vigilant and pay close attention to food labels. If you eat out often, you have to take extra care, since you do not have much control over what goes into the food you eat.

Very often during the first few days, you may find your symptoms becoming aggravated before they start to improve.

The challenging phase

If you find no improvement in your heartburn symptoms after 2 continuous weeks of the diet, it's time to consult your medical practitioner. Perhaps he or she may suggest alternative options.

If your symptoms are showing signs of improvement, it's time for a challenge. Introduce your body to the food items that you have eliminated one at a time. Start with a small portion in the morning. If you don't experience any heartburn, eat a larger amount at lunch and then again in the evening.

Add a new food group once every three days, so you can be sure the symptoms do not come back. Make a note of the symptoms.

If the food does not produce Acid Reflux symptoms during the three-day challenge, it is unlikely that it is a food offender. You can add this item back to your diet once you have tested all the other food items on your challenge list.

The reassessment phase

Now you have your elimination results in hand. The next step is to come up with an Acid Reflux diet that will help you to stay healthy and pain free. You must always remember that there are several other factors that can interfere with the effectiveness of this diet.

Be open to any new developments. And always pay attention to nutrition. Even if you need to give up one type of food, such as dairy— try to find other sources of calcium like almonds or leafy greens. You want to make sure that you are getting all the nutrients your body needs.

Always remember that patience and time are your two greatest allies when you are doing the elimination diet. You may need to try and try again, until you are able to identify the foods that may be causing problems. Continue reassessing your diet until all your symptoms have disappeared.

CHAPTER 6

Natural remedies to support your Acid Reflux Diet

The best way to deal with your Acid Reflux is to restore your natural gastric balance and function. In addition to making positive changes in your day-to-day diet and lifestyle, there are a number of strategies involving natural remedies which may help you get a grip on your GERD symptoms, sans medication.

Of late, many have been trying to avoid pharmaceuticals as much as possible and have been looking for an alternative way to reduce their symptoms and restore their body to its natural balance.

Though there hasn't been much research into herbal remedies for heartburn, many complementary and alternative medicine treatments have been tried. Some of them have been successful in providing relief to GERD symptoms as well as promote healing by calming your digestive system.

Your Acid Reflux diet is not about what you have to give up. Following such a diet should not make you feel like you are being punished or deprived.

If you would like to treat your conditions exclusively with non-medical therapies, here are some possible solutions, including some food items that act as digestion-aids:

Ginger.

Ginger is a delicious treat that can be added to many kinds of meals. It can also absorb stomach acid and calm your nerves. Ginger is a spice, a food, and has been used as a natural remedy with medicinal qualities for millennia. Scientists have performed numerous studies on its health benefits, and it has been evaluated for its usefulness in treating over 100 health conditions and diseases. It is truly one of the world's most versatile, evidence-based remedies.

Include fresh ginger to your Acid Reflux diet food, or enjoy it candied, pickled or dried. You can make yourself a cup of ginger tea.

Refreshing Ginger Tea

Serves 1

Ingredients:

2-3 slices fresh ginger   2 cups hot water
1 lemon

Method:

1. Juice the lemon.
2. Boil 2 cups of water. Add fresh ginger root slices into the hot water. Allow it to steep for about half an hour. Add in the lemon juice and drink about 20 minutes or so before your meal.

Fennel

Fennel is known to calm the process of digestion by suppressing stomach spasms and also hastening the movement of the food from the stomach to the intestine. Fennel works wonders for stomach bloating and digestion. Add it in your food while cooking or chew on some fennel after your meal. Fennel works as a great mouth freshener as well.

Apple Cider Vinegar

Apple cider vinegar contains enzymes that can prevent acid reflux. Add 3 teaspoons of raw unfiltered apple cider vinegar into 6 to 8 ounces of drinking water and drink it before your meals.

Baking soda

Baking Soda is known to ease the burn of acid reflux since it neutralizes the stomach acids. For quick relief, add one-half teaspoon of baking soda (sodium bicarbonate) in an 8-ounce glass of water.

However, overconsumption of baking soda can be detrimental to your health because it contains sodium which can raise your blood pressure and make your blood too alkaline. So, do not consume too much of it.

Probiotics

An imbalance of the bacteria in your gut or too little "good" bacteria in your gastrointestinal tract can compromise your ability to fight illness and disease. By taking probiotic supplements in the context of your Acid Reflux diet, you will be able to get back this balance.

Almonds

Almonds are known to neutralize your stomach acids and thus help to prevent or relieve your heartburn. Snack on 3 to 4 almonds as soon as you have eaten or use them in any of your Acid Reflux diet recipes. Here is a great breakfast idea using almonds. This delicious Acid Reflux diet-friendly breakfast recipe is filling, and will keep those mid-morning hunger pangs at bay.

Berry, nutty oatmeal

Serves: 4

Ingredients:

2 cups low-fat milk
¼ cup melted butter
1 tablespoon vanilla extract
1 cup old fashioned oats
½ cup chopped roasted almonds

½ cup dates
½ tsp baking powder
1 cup blueberries
1 cup chopped strawberries

Method:

1. Preheat oven to 375° F.
2. Whisk the low-fat milk, melted butter and vanilla together.
3. Spread a dab of butter evenly on the baking dish and place oats, roasted almonds, dates, and baking powder into it.
4. Pour the milk, butter and vanilla mixture over the ingredients and top with berries.
5. Bake for about 45 minutes or until liquid is absorbed.

Papaya and Pineapple

Papaya contains papain and pineapple contains bromelain, both of which are natural digestive enzymes that help with the breakdown of protein and reduce inflammation. Your body normally digests proteins using an enzyme called pepsin which works like a charm in the extremely acidic environment of the stomach. But when you are on an Acid Reflux diet that works on reducing your stomach acids, the proteins may not be digested properly. You will then experience heartburn and pain.

When you include papaya and pineapple to your Acid Reflux Diet, you help to facilitate the breakdown of proteins and therefore ease your heartburn symptoms. Here is a fantastic fruit smoothie that can help soothe your symptoms.

Heartburn smoothie

Serves: 2

Ingredients:

1 cup diced fresh papaya

1 cup diced fresh pineapple

½ cup Greek yogurt

½ cup ice

1 sprig of mint

½ cup water

Method:

1. Mix all the above ingredients into a blender.
2. Top with the sprig of mint and enjoy.

CHAPTER 7

What to avoid on an Acid Reflux Diet

We have discussed in the previous chapters that Acid Reflux may be triggered by different things for different people. But having said that, there are still some food and drinks which are more prone to allow your stomach's contents to splash up into your esophagus and cause GERD.

Let's call these food items the "recognized food offenders." Some of these food items may be among your favorites, but it is advisable to eat less of them so that you can prevent the uncomfortable feeling of heartburn from ever starting.

1. Spicy Food

It may be stating the obvious, but spicy food items are your enemies if you are looking to prevent heartburn. Some hot spices irritate the esophagus and cause Acid Reflux. It is best to avoid chili peppers and spicy seasonings and sauces.

If you really can't control your yearning for Thai or Indian food, request "no-spice" food. Very often, even the "mild" version of a Thai green curry, for example, may wreak havoc on your GERD. Avoiding hot spices will certainly help stave off those unbearable, painful symptoms and also reduce chances of your developing stomach ulcers.

If you just love Thai food but the spices and grease scare you, we have just the fix for you. Here is a clean and healthy Acid Reflux Diet version of Thai sweet and spicy pineapple fried rice—a quick weeknight dinner you can make in the comfort of your home.

Thai sweet and spicy pineapple fried rice

Serves: 2

Ingredients:

2 tablespoons coconut oil

2 eggs, beaten with a dash of salt

1 cup chopped fresh pineapple

½ bunch green onions, sliced

2 cloves garlic, pressed or minced

½ cup chopped raw, unsalted cashews

2 cups cooked brown jasmine rice

1 tablespoon soy sauce

1 small lime, halved

Sea salt, to taste

Small bunch of fresh cilantro leaves, chopped

Method:

1. Prepare all the ingredients and keep it ready before you start cooking. Leftover rice from the refrigerator works best as it is not sticky.
2. Heat oil in a large pan and add ½ tablespoon of oil. Break in the eggs and scramble them until they are cooked. Transfer the eggs to an empty bowl.
3. Add one tablespoon of oil into the same pan. Add the pineapple and stir constantly for about 3-5 minutes, until the pineapple juice evaporates, and the edges of the fruit have caramelized.
4. Add the sliced green onions and garlic.
5. Stir constantly and cook until fragrant. Now transfer this to your bowl of scrambled eggs.
6. Now, add the remaining ½ tablespoon of oil to the same pan. Add in the cashews and stir constantly, until the cashews are lightly browned.
7. Add the cooked rice to the pan and mix until the rice is hot.
8. Finally, add the contents of the bowl back into the pan and mix well. Remove the pan from heat. And add 1 tablespoon soy sauce and some sea salt to taste.
9. Squeeze out the juice of ½ of a lime over the rice and stir thoroughly.
10. Garnish with chopped cilantro and serve into individual serving bowls.

2. High Fat Food items

Food items that have high fat content may cause acid reflux. This is because fatty food items need a large amount of acid to digest. So the contents of your stomach become highly acidic. The food ends up sitting in your stomach for a longer time, causing a reflux.

Another reason why you get heartburn when you consume your favorite fatty treats could be because they may also cause a weakening of the lower esophageal sphincter. Trans fats have been linked to esophageal disease on many occasions, so any problems relating to the esophagus can also exacerbate your heartburn symptoms.

Since fried food items are high in fat content, it is advisable to avoid food that is fried in fat—both deep fried and shallow fried. This means bidding farewell to chips and fries and saying hello to baked sweet potato or zucchini wedges.

Golden sweet potato sticks

Serves: 2

Ingredients:

1 large sweet potato, peeled and cut into long wedges

2 tablespoons freshly ground flax seeds

Salt- to taste

Freshly ground pepper- to taste

Method:

1. Preheat the oven to 400° F.
2. Spray the baking dish with nonstick cooking spray.
3. Season the sweet potato with salt and pepper to taste.
4. Spread them in an even layer on a baking dish. Bake the potatoes for 10 minutes. Turn them over and bake again for 10 minutes.
5. Remove from the oven to a serving dish and sprinkle freshly ground flax seeds.

3. Alcoholic beverages

If you are suffering from Acid Reflux, it's about time to rethink your drinking. Alcohol is known to relax the sphincter as well as irritate the lining of the stomach. The higher the alcohol content in a beverage, the greater the damage. Drinks with lower alcohol content stimulate acid secretion in your stomach.

If you cannot abstain from consuming alcoholic beverages, indulge in them in moderation.

Go ahead, celebrate. A glass of red wine may not be a big deal on its own, but what you are eating to accompany it also matters. If you are dining out in an Italian restaurant, for example, and order spaghetti Napolitano as the main course, you are definitely inviting trouble, as the base of the Napolitano sauce is tomato, and tomato and heartburn are not the best of friends.

4. Chocolate and mint

If you are a chocoholic, sorry, I have bad news for you. Chocolate and mint have substances that can stimulate the release of stomach acids. They also tend to weaken the lower esophageal sphincter. Stay away from both.

5. High-fat dairy products

As discussed earlier, all high-fat food items cause heartburn, so this includes your favorite cheeses and butter. Instead, enjoy plant-based options like almond milk, coconut or soy yogurt. These options have lower amounts of unhealthy fats.

6. Coffee

Cut back on coffee. Besides decreasing pressure in the lower esophageal sphincter, the acidic nature of coffee also irritates your stomach. Enjoy mild green tea, chamomile tea or herbal teas instead.

7. Sodas

Most sodas contain caffeine and are very acidic in nature. Sodas don't help you in any way, and for most people, they simply satisfy a sugar addiction.

8. Spices and Chili peppers

Hot spices and chili peppers aggravate your heartburn. Avoid cayenne, chili, black pepper, mustard, cinnamon and nutmeg. That doesn't mean you have to settle for bland food.

Boost flavor and add character to your food using fresh herbs such as ginger, basil and cilantro. Dried herbs like thyme, rosemary, dill, and oregano can take your Acid Reflux Diet food from good to great.

CHAPTER 8

Cooking methods that keep heartburn pains at bay

Before we get to the recipes, let's discuss about how you can choose heartburn-friendly food and cook a healthy meal that does not produce reflux symptoms. Sometimes, it's not only what you eat that gives you Acid Reflux but also how the food is cooked.

Cooking techniques can cause excessive secretion of the hormone gastrin, which in turn triggers production of stomach acid. A simple switch in your preparation technique can greatly reduce the severity and frequency of GERD.

Forget frying.

Satisfy your craving for fried food items using cooking techniques that imitate them. If you are yearning to get your hands on a bucket of fried chicken, look for alternative recipes which create a similar crispy texture and flavor with less risk of aggravating your heartburn. The crispy baked chicken we discuss below may look and taste exactly like fried chicken, but it will also save you from lots of pain and discomfort.

Try your hand at baking instead.

Whether you suffer from GERD or not, baking may be one of the healthiest methods of food preparation. Your food is cooked by surrounding it with hot air from all sides in your oven. You don't need to add much fat to your cooking either.

Crispy baked chicken

Serves: 2

Ingredients:

4 pieces boneless, skinless chicken breasts

1 cup chicken broth

1 cup bread crumbs

Salt to taste

Pepper to taste

Directions:

1. Preheat the oven to 350° F.
2. Spray a baking sheet with olive oil.
3. Mix together the breadcrumbs, salt and pepper on another plate.
4. Coat each chicken piece with chicken broth and then drag it through the breadcrumb mixture.
5. Place each piece of chicken on the baking sheet. Bake at 350° F for 12 to 15 minutes. Serve immediately.

Get ready to fire up the grill.

Grilling is a dry cooking method which reduces the total fat of whatever it is you're fixing. The fat gets melted and drips away from the meat. Grill lean meat, like turkey tenders or chicken thighs. Brush the meat with some mild teriyaki or barbecue sauce and enjoy the smoky flavors created by grilling.

Grilled Teriyaki chicken with pineapple

Serves: 2

Ingredients:

2 boneless skinless chicken breasts

3 tablespoons brown sugar

3 tablespoons soy sauce

1 tablespoon cornstarch

1 tablespoon water

1 cup fresh pineapple chunks

2 garlic cloves, minced

Pepper to taste

Salt to taste

Sliced green onions, for garnish

Roasted sesame seeds, for garnish

Method:

1. Whisk together the brown sugar, soy sauce, garlic, pepper, and salt in a sauce pan. Mix water and cornstarch separately and add to the brown sugar and soy sauce mixture.
2. Bring the sauce to boil and boil about 1-3 minutes. When the sauce starts to thicken, remove from heat. Keep aside a small amount for brushing.
3. Marinate the chicken breasts in the sauce and refrigerate for at least 30 minutes.
4. Grill the chicken evenly on both sides for 6-7 minutes.
5. Grill the pineapple chunks lightly.
6. Serve the grilled chicken and the pineapple on the plate and brush with sauce before serving.
7. Garnish with green onion and sprinkle roasted sesame seeds.

Steam it up.

Steaming is a great way to bring out the flavor of vegetables and seafood. Since it retains the form and texture of the vegetable or fish, without adding any fat, it is a perfect method of cooking for Acid Reflux.

Choose a convenient steamer for your kitchen; it could be either an electric steamer, a Chinese bamboo steamer inserted into a wok or a covered, perforated basket which is placed over a pot of boiling water.

You could also choose to steam your fish or tender vegetables in foil or parchment paper, adding in some flavorful liquid like broth or lemon juice. Place the wrapped food into the oven. The liquid converts to steam in the hot oven and quickly cooks all the ingredients.

Steamed dilled salmon in a bed of leeks

Serves: 2

Ingredients:

2 salmon fillets
½ teaspoon dried dill
1 bunch leeks
2 teaspoons olive oil

Salt to taste
Tarragon to taste
2 teaspoons Dijon mustard

Method:

1. Preheat oven to 425° F.
2. Rinse the leeks after removing the dark-green tops and root ends. Slice them lengthwise in halves and again into quarters.
3. Place 2 pieces of foil, approximately 12" x 12" each on counter and lay half the leeks in the center. Pour 1 teaspoon of olive oil on the leeks. Sprinkle tarragon and salt to taste.
4. Place the salmon fillet on top of the leeks and spread the Dijon mustard.
5. Sprinkle dill.
6. Cover the fish by folding in all the sides of the foil and create a tightly sealed packet.
7. Place on a baking sheet and bake for 20 minutes.
8. When done, transfer sealed packages to your dinner plates and open before you are ready to eat.
9. Serve with brown rice.

Relish your roasts.

Food items are roasted by cooking them in an uncovered pan. This method of dry cooking may not be suited to break down tougher fibers but is a perfect way to cook tender meats.

A delicious, caramelized flavor is brought out in meats and vegetables. Ensure you use an open, large pan which allows the moisture to escape quickly. If not, the moisture will prevent the food from having a crusty brown exterior.

Roasted Root Vegetables

Serves: 2

Ingredients:

1 tablespoon olive oil

4 red potatoes, cubed

4 carrots, peeled and cut into 1 inch pieces

4 parsnips, peeled and cut into 1 inch pieces

2 teaspoons dried rosemary

Salt to taste

Freshly ground black pepper to taste

Method:

1. Preheat the oven to 350°F. Add olive oil in a large roasting pan in the oven and add the potatoes, carrots, parsnips, rosemary, salt and pepper. Ensure all the vegetables are coated with the oil. Stir gently every 10 minutes and roast for about 20 to 30 minutes.

Cooking under pressure

Pressure cooking is a quick method of cooking food that uses minimum water and no fat and produces boiled, stewed or poached food items. This is one of the best ways to cook Acid Reflux recipes because you can cook without adding fat and retain all the nutrients in your food.

To pressure cook, you add the food that's in a closed container into another pot that uses steam and pressure to increase the temperature.

Yellow mung beans kedgeree

Serves: 2

Ingredients:

½ cup split yellow mung beans

½ cup brown basmati rice

1 teaspoon ghee

1 teaspoon black mustard seeds

½ teaspoon cumin

1 teaspoon fenugreek seeds

1 pinch asafetida

1 teaspoon crushed fresh ginger root

½ teaspoon turmeric powder

2 bay leaves

2 cups water

Fresh cilantro, chop and garnish

Salt to taste

Method:

1. Wash the mung beans and rice together, rubbing them between your fingers. Wash until the water runs clear. Soak for 3-4 hours.
2. Heat ghee in the pressure cooker and add the mustard. Wait until the mustard seeds pop.
3. Pop in fenugreek seeds, cumin and a pinch of asafetida.
4. Add some ginger and turmeric powder, salt to taste and finally the mung beans and rice. Mix well until the rice and beans are coated with the spice mixture.

5. Add the water and bay leaves to the rice and bean mixture and close the pressure cooker. Pressure cook for 10- 15 minutes.

6. Serve with chopped cilantro.

CHAPTER 9

Breakfast Recipes

When you wake up in the morning, your stomach is pretty much empty. Breakfast, the first meal of the day, provides your body with a much needed source of fuel to get you revved up for the day ahead. It is always beneficial to avoid having an empty stomach, whether you have Acid Reflux or not.

Did your mother ever tell you to "Eat breakfast like a king?" Well, mothers are usually right. But remember, at the same time, eating a lot can provoke reflux.

An ideal breakfast for someone with Acid Reflux would be a well-balanced carb-intensive one with the proper mix of proteins. Very often, fast food breakfasts include a lot of baked items that are high in sugar and fat—think cream cheese bagels, donuts and muffins. These items may be about as healthy as cupcakes are—minus the layer of frosting.

The key to successfully keeping your Acid Reflux under control is proper planning. Stock your pantry and your refrigerator with the right ingredients for a healthy heartburn free breakfast. Here are some breakfast suggestions that are not too light and not too large.

Tofu and mushroom scramble

Serves: 2

Ingredients:

8 oz. extra firm tofu
1 tablespoon olive oil
½ lb mushrooms
1 cup baby spinach, shredded
½ red onion

1 pinch turmeric
Freshly ground black pepper to taste
Salt to taste
2 basil leaves

Method:

1. Crumble the tofu in your hands over a bowl.
2. Now chop and fry the onion in a pan.

3. Dice the mushrooms into halves and add them to the onions.
4. Throw in shredded spinach and add a pinch of turmeric.
5. Add in the pepper and salt to taste.
6. Cook until the tofu has warmed up.
7. Finally throw in the torn basil leaves and serve it on toasted, sprouted bread.

Flavorful farmer's market omelet

Serves: 2

Ingredients:

3 eggs

¼ cup water

2 ounces fat-free feta cheese, crumbled

½ teaspoon dried basil leaves

¼ teaspoon garlic powder

2 teaspoons butter

For the filling:

1 cup baby spinach

¼ cup thinly sliced yellow summer squash

¼ cup thinly sliced zucchini

¼ cup chopped red bell pepper

2 tablespoons water

Method:

1. Heat a pan and cook all the filling ingredients with 2 tablespoons of water over medium heat. Keep stirring. Remove from heat when the water has evaporated and vegetables are cooked. Keep the vegetables aside.
2. Beat eggs with ¼ cup water, cheese, basil and garlic powder.
3. Heat butter, and coat the base of the pan. Pour half of the egg mixture into the pan.
4. Gently move the cooked portions from the edge of the pan towards the center. Tilt the pan and move the uncooked portions so it can cook.
5. When the upper surface of the eggs have thickened and no visible liquid egg remains, place half of the filling on one side of the omelet. Fold the omelet in half and slide onto plate.
6. Make the second omelet by repeating the steps above.
7. Serve immediately.

Nutty banana split with yogurt and honey

Serves: 1

Ingredients:

1 ripe banana, peeled
½ cup Greek yogurt
1 tablespoon honey

2 tablespoons sliced almonds, pistachio and walnuts
¼ cup fresh seasonal berries, like blackberries or raspberries

Method:

1. Split the banana lengthwise. Lay the two halves in a banana split boat or any shallow bowl.
2. Now, place the Greek yogurt over the banana.
3. Using a spoon, drizzle honey over the yogurt and sprinkle the nuts over it.
4. Top with the fresh seasonal berries.

Apple pancakes

Serves: 2

Ingredients:

1 tablespoon butter
1 tablespoon brown sugar
2 eggs
1 ½ cups flour
1 cup milk

1 teaspoon baking powder
1 cup finely diced apples
1/8 teaspoon cinnamon
1/8 teaspoon salt
Olive oil spray

Method:

1. Mix butter and brown sugar in a bowl and cream it thoroughly.
2. Whisk the eggs and add to butter and brown sugar mixture.
3. Separately, add the cinnamon to the flour and sift together. Now, mix the flour and cinnamon with the butter and sugar mixture.
4. Add finely diced apples. Blend well.
5. Now, pour milk into this mixture and mix until you have a medium-consistency batter.

6. Heat a lightly oiled non-stick frying pan over low heat. Pour 1/4 cup of apple mixture into it and gently spread it out into a round shape with the back of a spoon. Allow it to cook for 2 minutes. Turn over, and remove when cooked.

Baked Oatmeal

Serves: 2

Ingredients:

1 cups rolled oats (not quick cooking)
¼ cup raisins
1/8 cup brown sugar
½ teaspoon baking powder
1/8 teaspoon cinnamon
¼ cup applesauce

¼ cup yogurt
¼ cup milk
2 tablespoons butter
2 eggs
Salt to taste

Method:

1. Mix oats, raisins, brown sugar, baking powder, cinnamon, and salt together in a bowl.
2. Whisk the applesauce, yogurt, milk, butter, and eggs separately in another bowl.
3. Mix both the mixtures together.
4. Pour into greased baking pan and refrigerate overnight.
5. Bake at 350°F for 45-50 minutes.
6. Sprinkle brown sugar over the baked oatmeal and serve.

Breakfast casserole with spinach, cheese & mushrooms

Serves: 2

Ingredients:

3 tablespoons extra-virgin olive oil
1 cup bread, cut into 1-inch cubes
½ cup fresh mushrooms, sliced
2 cloves garlic, minced
¼ teaspoon fresh thyme leaves, roughly chopped

1 cup baby spinach
½ cup cheese, shredded
4 eggs
1 cup milk
Salt to taste
Freshly ground black pepper to taste

Method:

1. Coat a casserole dish with a little olive oil.
2. In a large bowl, toss the bread cubes with 2 tablespoons oil and salt and pepper to taste. Heat a pan over medium heat and add the bread cubes and toast until golden brown. Move this to a bowl to cool.
3. Wipe out the pan and heat the remaining oil over medium-high heat. Spread the mushrooms well to form a layer and cook until they are brown.
4. Add the minced garlic, thyme and salt and pepper to taste. Stir continuously for a minute. Pop in the spinach. Cook until the spinach is wilted, while stirring continuously.
5. Place half the bread cubes in the prepared casserole dish, and sprinkle half of the cheese on top of it. Next, add the mushroom-spinach mixture in an even layer.
6. Now top with the remaining bread cubes and cheese.
7. Whisk together the eggs and milk with some salt and pepper in another bowl and pour it into the casserole dish.
8. Cover with cling wrap, and refrigerate overnight or for at least 6 hours.
9. Take the casserole out of the refrigerator half an hour before baking.
10. Preheat the oven to 350° F. Bake for 50 to 55 minutes until the top is golden brown.
11. Serve when cooled to room temperature.

CHAPTER 10

Lunch Recipes

Lunching out can be one of the major triggers for people suffering from Acid Reflux. The ready-to-eat greasy and high-fat food items you end up eating in restaurants and fast food outlets stay in your stomach for a long time and encourage the production of excessive stomach acids. Brown bagging your meals to take to work or eating at home will reduce your chances of triggering your Acid Reflux symptoms for a very simple reason—you control what goes into your food.

If you are unable to avoid eating out for lunch, start packing your own meals instead. Include some lighter, easy to digest food items like a fresh salad and some lean turkey sandwiches in whole wheat bread and some Greek yogurt topped with berries for a nutritionally well-balanced, easy-to-digest meal.

Sure, this will require some planning, and stocking up your refrigerator and pantry with food items that won't provoke heartburn symptoms. Here are some ideas that will keep that burning sensation at bay whether you are having lunch at home or at work. These dishes can be made quickly and easily.

To spend less time in the kitchen, try doubling these recipes. You can then reheat them later in the week. Instead of relying on convenience food items, always cook from scratch. This way, you know what you are really eating, and you are also able to control heartburn flare-ups effectively.

Tuna casserole

Serves: 2

Ingredients:

2 oz egg noodles
7 oz tuna, in water
½ cup frozen peas, thawed
12 oz can cream of mushroom soup, reduced fat
¼ cup plain yogurt, preferably fat-free
½ cup milk, preferably fat-free

1 tablespoon Dijon mustard
Pepper to taste
1/8 teaspoon dried basil
1 oz shredded cheddar
½ oz crushed, potato chips, baked
Fresh parsley, for garnish

Method:

1. Boil noodles.
2. Drain tuna and flake the meat.
3. Mix the soup, yogurt, milk and mustard together in a bowl.
4. Add the tuna and peas and mix.
5. Move this mixture into a baking dish, and gently stir in noodles.
6. Sprinkle the cheese and chips over the dish.
7. Bake at 350° F for 30 minutes.
8. Sprinkle some chopped fresh parsley over the dish.

Shrimp and vegetables stir-fry

Serves: 2

Ingredients:

2 tablespoons olive oil

½ cup raw medium peeled shrimp

½ cup broccoli florets

½ cups sliced mushrooms

1 scallion, trimmed and chopped

½ tablespoon garlic, minced

½ tablespoon fresh ginger, minced

½ cup cold vegetable broth mixed with

1 tablespoon cornstarch

Salt- to taste

1 cup organic millet or brown rice

Method:

1. Heat oil till it reaches its smoking point in a pan or wok.
2. Add broccoli, mushroom, ginger, garlic and scallions and stir constantly till al dente.
3. Add shrimp and continue to stir until it turns pink.
4. Add some salt to taste and cover until shrimp has cooked.
5. Add cornstarch and broth mixture. Keep stirring until it thickens.
6. Remove from heat and serve over millet or brown rice cooked according to instructions on the pack.

Chicken Salad with ginger and sesame

Serves: 2

Ingredients:

1 large chicken breast, diced

3 teaspoons light soy sauce

2 teaspoons sesame oil

1 teaspoon fresh grated ginger

¼ teaspoon ground coriander

¼ teaspoon rice vinegar

3 cups baby spinach

12 baby carrots, halved

¼ cup sliced almonds, toasted

1 tablespoon sesame seeds, toasted

1 teaspoon olive oil

Method:

1. Make the marinade by mixing the soy sauce, sesame oil, ginger, and coriander and rice vinegar together in a bowl.
2. Dice the chicken and coat thoroughly with the marinade. Move this to the refrigerator and keep for at least 1 hour in the fridge.
3. Heat a nonstick pan over medium-high and add chicken to the pan. Stir-fry until cooked.
4. Place the spinach and carrots in 2 salad bowls. Drizzle with vinegar and olive oil, and top with chicken.
5. Sprinkle toasted almonds and sesame seeds over the salad for that extra crunch.

Mushroom and bean burgers

Serves: 4

Ingredients:

1 15 oz can kidney beans, drained and rinsed

1 tablespoon olive oil

½ teaspoon soy sauce

2 cups sliced mushrooms

¼ cup slivered almonds

1 small carrot, grated

½ cup whole-wheat breadcrumbs

1 egg white

2 tablespoons chopped fresh parsley

½ teaspoon ground coriander

½ teaspoon dried oregano

½ teaspoon ground ginger

Salt to taste

Method:

1. Heat olive oil in a pan and add sliced mushrooms to it. Stir occasionally until it has browned. Put aside to cool.
2. Cook the beans in a pressure cooker for 5 minutes. If you do not have a pressure cooker, microwave for 5 minutes. Smash with a fork until it has a nearly smooth consistency. Add the olive oil, soy sauce, browned mushrooms,

almonds, grated carrot, half the breadcrumbs, egg white, oregano, ginger, parsley and coriander. Add salt to taste. Mix with your hands until it has reached a uniform consistency.

3. Spread the remaining breadcrumbs onto a plate. Shape the bean mixture into 4 patties and lightly coat with the breadcrumbs, making sure to dust off any excess.
4. Add some cooking spray to a large nonstick pan over medium heat. Cook the patties until golden and slightly crisp.
5. Serve the patties in whole-wheat burger buns or over salad greens.

Veggie sandwich with hummus and avocado paste

Serves: 1

Ingredients:

2 slices of whole-grain bread
2 small carrots, thinly sliced on a heavy angle
¼ of an avocado

1 tablespoon hummus
1/8 teaspoon dried oregano
Pepper to taste
Handful of baby spinach

Method:

1. Toast the bread.
2. In the meantime, peel the carrots and slice them finely on a heavy angle.
3. Spread avocado on one piece of toast and hummus on the other piece. Sprinkle oregano and pepper on the hummus.
4. Layer the carrots and spinach on one slice of the bread, and cover with the other.
5. Cut it in half and serve with any remaining spinach or carrot slices on the side.

Green beans with sesame

Serves: 4

Ingredients:

1 lb. green beans, trimmed

1 tablespoon soy sauce

½ teaspoon ginger root, freshly grated

¼ tablespoon butter

2 teaspoons sesame seeds, toasted

1 tablespoon rice wine vinegar

Salt to taste

Method:

1. Steam green beans in a steamer until they are cooked but still crisp.
2. Place in a serving bowl and add all the other ingredients. Toss well and serve with brown rice.

Char grilled chicken with tahini dressing

Serves: 2

Ingredients:

1 cup quinoa

½ cucumber, cut into 1-inch chunks

4 cherry tomatoes, halved

2 spring onions, finely sliced

2 tablespoons olive oil

½ lemon, juiced

Handful parsley, roughly chopped

Handful coriander, roughly chopped

2 chicken breasts

Ingredients for the tahini dressing

1½ tablespoons tahini paste (Paste made from ground sesame seeds, often used in Middle Eastern cooking and found in speciality shops and larger supermarkets.)

1½ tablespoon low-fat yogurt

½ lemon, juice

½ garlic clove, crushed

½ teaspoons forest honey

3 tablespoons water

Method:

1. Rinse the quinoa into a saucepan and pour in 2 cups of water. Cover the container and allow it to boil. Reduce heat and simmer until the water has evaporated. Put it aside, and let it cool.
2. Place the cucumber, cherry tomatoes, spring onions and herbs into a salad bowl. Add 1 tablespoon olive oil and lemon juice and mix well.
3. Rub the chicken breasts with 1 tablespoon olive oil. Heat a non-stick pan and fry on both sides until cooked.
4. Stir together the tahini paste, yogurt, lemon juice, garlic and honey with 3 tablespoons of water to form the tahini dressing.
5. Toss the quinoa together with the salad and place on plates.
6. Place the chicken on the quinoa and drizzle the dressing over it.

Turkey & asparagus with melted cheese

Serves: 2

Ingredients:

4 oz asparagus, trimmed and cut into 1-inch pieces

1/3 cup chicken broth

1 teaspoon plus 2 tablespoons all-purpose flour, keep separate

2 boneless, skinless turkey breasts

Salt to taste

Freshly ground pepper to taste

1 tablespoon olive oil

1 shallot, thinly sliced

¼ cup white wine

¼ cup sour cream

1 teaspoon chopped fresh tarragon

1 teaspoon lemon juice

½ cup shredded cheese

Method:

1. Steam the asparagus in a steamer. If you don't have a steamer, place a perforated basket in a large pot and add 1 inch of water and bring to a boil. Place the asparagus in the perforated basket, cover and steam for 3 minutes. Remove from the heat and put aside.
2. Mix the chicken broth and 1 teaspoon flour in a small bowl until smooth. Put aside.
3. Put the remaining 2 tablespoons of flour into a flat dish. Sprinkle the turkey with salt and pepper and pat both sides in the flour. Dust off any excess flour.
4. Heat oil in a large pan and add the chicken. Cook until golden brown on both sides. Move to a plate and cover to keep warm.

5. Add shallot, wine and the broth and flour mixture to the pan and cook over medium heat. Keep stirring continuously until it thickens.
6. Bring the heat down to medium-low. Add the tarragon, sour cream and lemon juice.
7. Now place the turkey into the pan and mix well so that the sauce coats the entire surface of the meat.
8. Add the steamed asparagus.
9. Add cheese over the turkey breasts and cook until the cheese has melted.
10. Serve hot.

CHAPTER 11

Dinner Recipes

Nighttime reflux can be troublesome. In order to control nighttime reflux, you should plan to finish dinner by 8 p.m., or at a time that's at least three to four hours before going to sleep. This also means avoiding snacking of any kind. Yes, for many of us, eating dinner early represents a significant lifestyle shift. It means eating well-planned breakfasts, lunches and snacks. It also means making healthy food and beverage choices.

Everyone enjoys a drink at dinner, but we know that drinking alcohol may be an Acid Reflux trigger. Limiting your alcohol intake at dinner time can help a great deal in controlling nighttime reflux.

A kitchen cooking Acid Reflux meals is not complete without a large and small non-stick skillet. These skillets will allow you to cook many of your favorite food items without having to add as much fat. Here are some delicious, nutritious dinner options that are low on fat and light on your stomach.

Nourishing vegetable soup

Serves: 4

Ingredients:

1 small zucchini, chopped
1 cup beetroot, chopped
½ cup carrots, peeled and chopped
1 small onion
Sprig of parsley

½ cup pearl barley, rinsed
6 cups distilled water
2 celery stalks, stocks chopped and leaves reserved

Method:

1. Bring the distilled water to boil in a large soup pot.
2. Chop all vegetables into very fine pieces and add to water.
3. Add barley and simmer, partially covered, for 40 minutes.

4. Stir in the chopped celery leaves into soup. Serve with whole wheat dinner rolls.

Spinach soup with cheddar

Serves: 4

Ingredients:

1 tablespoon olive oil

5 oz spinach, washed

1 clove garlic, finely minced

2 tablespoons butter

1 small Onion

1/8 cup flour

2 cups milk

Salt to taste

Black pepper to taste

4 oz cheddar, extra-sharp, grated

Method:

1. Heat 1 tablespoon olive oil in an iron skillet over medium heat.
2. Add spinach and garlic and cook until the spinach wilts.
3. Add spinach to a blender with ¼ cup hot water and puree. Put this aside.
4. Heat butter in a large soup pot, and add chopped onion.
5. When the onion has softened, sprinkle flour on it and stir to combine.
6. Pour in milk and stir continuously.
7. Add salt and pepper, and mix.
8. While stirring constantly, cook the sauce over medium heat for 5 minutes.
9. Pour in pureed spinach and the grated cheese. Continue stirring until the cheese has melted.
10. Serve in a bowl. Add a little grated cheese on top as a garnish.

Cheesy butternut squash

Serves: 4

Ingredients:

1 large butternut squash

1 teaspoon olive oil

2 tablespoons grated white cheddar

Salt to taste

Pepper to taste

Fresh parsley, for garnish

Method:

1. Preheat the oven to 375° F. Coat a casserole dish with olive oil spray.
2. Remove the skin from the butternut squash and slice it in half. Remove the seeds and cut into 2-inch cubes.
3. Toss butternut squash chunks with olive oil in the casserole dish. Add salt and pepper to taste. Toss well.
4. Bake for 30 minutes at 375° F. Remove the casserole from the oven.
5. Stir the squash, and return it to the oven. Bake the squash for 15 minutes more or until squash is tender and lightly browned.
6. Remove squash from the oven and sprinkle with white cheddar cheese. Garnish with parsley and serve.

Delightful Roasted Vegetables

Serves: 4

Ingredients:

½ butternut squash, peeled and cut into 2-inch cubes

1 medium-sized eggplant, cut into 2-inch chunks

1 bunch asparagus, ends cut off and cut into 2-inch pieces

1 whole red onion, peeled and cut into 2-inch chunks

1 red bell pepper, seeded and cut into 2-inch pieces

2 parsnips, cut into 2-inch pieces

8 oz mushrooms, halved

3 cloves garlic, minced

2 sprigs of fresh rosemary

Salt to taste

Pepper to taste

3 tablespoons olive oil

Method

1. Preheat oven to 375° F.
2. Put all the prepped veggies in a large bowl with the minced garlic.
3. Break off the rosemary over the veggies and drizzle in the olive oil and allow it to spread throughout. Add salt and pepper to taste. Toss to coat all the vegetables evenly.
4. Lay out the vegetables on a baking sheet and put it into the preheated oven for 40 minutes.
5. Stir every 15 minutes or so for thorough roasting.
6. Serve immediately.

Sautéed white fish with mashed potatoes and greens

Serves: 1

Method:

1 4 oz filet of white fish (sole, flounder, etc.)

1 potato

1 tablespoon heavy cream

1 tablespoon milk

1 cup steamed green vegetable such as spinach, carrot, broccoli or peas

Parsley, for garnish

1 tablespoon butter

Method:

Mashed potatoes:

1. Peel potato and cut into 1-inch cubes. Place in a pan with cold water to cover, and bring to boil until cooked.
2. Drain. Leave just enough water in the potato for mashing. Add salt to taste.
3. Put the potato back on low heat and mash for 2 to 3 minutes. Turn off heat, and then add half tablespoon butter, milk, heavy cream, salt and pepper.

Fish:

1. Season fish with salt and pepper to taste. Place your large skillet over medium high heat. Add the remaining half tablespoon butter and then add fish.
2. Cook for two minutes on one side until light brown and cooked through. Turn and cook other side.
3. Serve fish over mashed potatoes. Place the steamed vegetables by the side of the fish. Garnish with chopped parsley.

Old-fashioned stew

Serves: 4

Ingredients:

2 tablespoons olive oil

½ pound beef stew meat

2 slices turkey bacon, chopped

1 medium sized onion, coarsely chopped

2 oz tomato paste

2 cups lower sodium beef broth

2 carrots, peeled and cut into 1-inch cubes

1 celery stalk, cut into 1-inch pieces

1 turnip, cut into 1-inch cubes

1 tablespoon fresh parsley, minced

1 tablespoon white vinegar

1 bay leaf

¼ teaspoon sugar

Salt and pepper to taste

Method:

1. On medium-high heat, add olive oil to a large heavy pot (use one with a tight fitting lid). Add bacon and cook until browned.
2. Add beef to the pot and add the salt and pepper when the beef browns. Stir occasionally.
3. Once browned, remove the meat from the pot using a slotted spoon and set aside.
4. Add onions into the pot. Sauté until it softens, and then add the tomato paste and vinegar. Cook for 5 minutes.
5. Now, pour in the beef broth, bay leaf, sugar and browned beef mixture. Stir constantly. Cover and cook on very low heat for about 45 minutes.
6. Add turnips, carrots, and celery, and simmer covered until the meat and vegetables are tender.
7. Taste and adjust salt and pepper as needed. Make sure that the sauce is thick. In case it is too thick, add in some beef broth until its consistency is just thin enough.
8. Discard the bay leaf and garnish with minced parsley.
9. Serve piping hot in a bowl with crusty bread or whole grain buns.

Roasted chicken with mushrooms and spinach

Serves: 2

Ingredients:

1 8oz. whole skinless, boneless chicken breast

1 cup cooked chickpeas

4 tablespoons olive oil

2 shallots, halved

2 garlic cloves, sliced thin

2 cups button mushrooms, sliced

1 pound of fresh spinach

½ lemon, juice

Salt to taste

Method:

1. Preheat the oven to 350°F.
2. Heat 2 tablespoons of olive oil in a cast-iron or regular ovenproof skillet on the stove over medium heat. Place the chicken in the hot oil, sprinkle salt and cook for about 5 minutes until brown on all sides.
3. Add the shallots and move the skillet to the oven and cook until the chicken is well done. Remove from the oven and put aside.
4. While the chicken is in the oven, heat 2 tablespoons of olive oil in another large skillet over medium-high heat and add the garlic. Once the garlic is fragrant, throw in the mushrooms and toss often to avoid sticking. Toss until the mushroom has cooked, then add the cooked chickpeas and stir well.
5. Place the spinach into the pan and cook until it wilts. Add salt to taste.
6. Divide the vegetable mixture on two dinner plates. Slice the chicken and serve over the vegetables. Squeeze some lemon over the chicken and serve.

Roasted turkey with warm corn & potato salad

Serves: 3

Ingredients:

1 lb turkey breasts (boneless and skinless)
2 strips turkey bacon
1 clove garlic
1 medium-sized bay leaf
1 small stick cinnamon
3 tablespoons olive oil
Crushed black pepper to taste
½ teaspoon brown sugar

Salt to taste
6 tiny new potatoes
1 large corn cob
½ red onion, thinly sliced
1 lime, juiced
1 tablespoon coriander leaves, roughly chopped

Method:

1. Cut the turkey breasts into 1-inch steaks. Sprinkle salt, pepper and brown sugar.
2. Warm 2 tablespoons olive oil in a large non-stick skillet over medium-high heat and add garlic, bay leaf, cinnamon stick, bacon strips and turkey steaks to the pan when the oil is hot. Cook the meat until golden brown on all sides.
3. Remove from heat and transfer the turkey to a shallow bowl. Cover the bowl tightly and leave for at least 10 minutes.

4. After it has cooled, cut each breast into ¼ inch slices. Remove the garlic, bay leaf, cinnamon stick and bacon and discard.

5. Boil water in a saucepan and cook the potatoes for 12 minutes. Add the corn after 6 minutes and remove from heat when both are cooked tender. Drain the water.

6. Mix the sliced red onion with the lime juice and 1 tablespoon olive oil in a large salad bowl. Add the boiled potatoes.

7. Stand the corn cob on one end on a chopping board. Slice down the length of it and cut the kernels from top to bottom and repeat all the way around the cob. Mix into the potato salad.

8. Sprinkle the coriander leaves, salt and pepper and serve alongside the roast turkey breast.

Steamed red snapper with spring onion & ginger

Serves: 2

Ingredients:

1 pound firm red snapper
2-inch piece fresh ginger, peeled and finely julienned
2 garlic cloves, finely sliced
2 tablespoons low-salt soy sauce

1 tablespoon rice wine
1 bunch spring onions, finely shredded
Small bunch cilantro, chopped
Salt to taste
White pepper to taste

Method:

1. Wash the fish in cold water. Pat dry with paper towels.

2. Season the fish with salt and pepper inside and out. Place some ginger inside the cavity of the fish and spread some on the skin.

3. Lay the remaining ginger in a shallow pan with the garlic, cilantro and spring onions. Place the fish on this bed.

4. Now pour over the soy sauce and rice wine, then season with salt and white pepper.

5. Add 2" of water into a large pot cover and boil. When the water has boiled, uncover and wipe the inside of the lid clean of any condensation so that it doesn't drip back down on your fish and dilute the flavor.

6. Put your fish pan inside, supported on a small inverted bowl so that it is not in direct contact with the boiling water.

7. Steam the fish on medium heat for about 12 minutes.

8. Serve with brown rice.

Conclusion

Thank you again for downloading this book!

I hope this book was able to help you to understand how you can control your Acid Reflux symptoms, improve your health and assist your body in achieving good digestive health.

GERD symptoms and conditions are unique to individuals based on body type, histories, allergies and physical conditioning. Successes always vary.

So, it is up it's you to discover the truth behind Acid Reflux and be your own advocates. The diet and lifestyle guidelines recommended in this book will help you overcome the symptoms and ultimately cure your heartburn and GERD. Don't allow Acid Reflux to take over your life.

Finally, if you enjoyed this book, then I'd like to ask you for a favor, would you be kind enough to leave a review for this book on Amazon? It'd be greatly appreciated!

Be sure to check out our website at www.thetotalevolution.com for more information.

Thank you and good luck!